Stretching & Massage

For hikers & backpackers

Victoria and Frank Logue
photos by Frank and Griffin Logue

Wilderness Press Berkeley, California

Photos by Frank and Griffin Logue
Cover and book design by Jaan Hitt

Library of Congress Card Number 2001046777
ISBN 0-89997-301-9

Manufactured in the United States of America

Published by Wilderness Press
        1200 Fifth Street
        Berkeley, CA 94710
        (800) 443-7227; FAX (510) 558-1696
        mail@wildernesspress.com
        www.wildernesspress.com

Contact us for a free catalog

Printed on recycled paper, 20% post-consumer waste

Library of Congress Cataloging-in-Publication Data
Logue, Victoria, 1961 -
Stretching & massage for hikers & backpackers / Victoria and
Frank Logue; photos by Frank and Griffin Logue.— 2nd ed.
    p. cm.
ISBN 0-89997-301-9
1. Hiking injuries—Prevention. 2. Backpacking injuries—
Prevention. 3. Stretching exercises. 4. Massage. I. Title:
Stretching and massage for hikers and backpackers. II. Logue,
Frank, 1963- III. Title.

RC88.9.H55 L64 2001
615.8'2—dc2I

                                            2001046777

Contents

Stretching continued

Massage

*Used together,
stretching and massage
will help your body heal itself*

Introduction

*L*et's face it, sometimes backpacking hurts. After a day of climbing and descending trails, your muscles can feel stiff and sore. But they don't have to. There is a drug-free way to reduce the aches and pains associated with backpacking. By stretching before you hit the trail and combining stretching and massage after hiking, you can help your body heal itself naturally.

The eleven stretches in this book will limber the areas that hikers and backpackers use most—the legs, the back, and the shoulders. This 15-minute routine of partner stretches will help prepare your body for hiking by stretching your muscles and increasing blood flow to these areas. After a hike, these stretches will help your body recover.

The eleven partner-massage techniques and three self-massage techniques in this book will help your body recover more quickly from the daily stress and strain of hiking and backpacking. Massage provides numerous benefits by wringing the toxins out of the blood stream and making way for oxygen-rich blood.

Always begin your stretching routine with a warm up

Stretching

*I*n the field of sports, backpacking is the only endurance sport in which participants do not regularly perform a stretching routine. Distance cyclists and marathon runners have long benefited from regular stretching before and after workouts. A proper stretching routine reduces the risk of muscle injury and increases flexibility over time. "Muscles or joints that lack adequate flexibility are more susceptible to injury," says Dr. Frank C. McCue III, Director of the Sports Medicine Division of the University of Virginia Health Sciences Center. "Good flexibility can prevent injury and enhance performance."

You should always begin your stretching routine with a warm-up. Studies show that stretching cold muscles does not improve flexibility and can lead to increased injuries. Five-to-ten minutes of aerobic exercise are enough to increase your heart rate and blood circulation to your muscles. You only need to begin to break a light sweat and noticeably breath heavier to be adequately warmed up. A brisk walk or slow jog will do the trick and make your stretching routine safer and more effective. An alternative is to stretch at your first rest stop of the day, when your body is already warmed up from hiking. If you do not have time to warm up, then forgo stretching.

Stretching at the end of the day is equally important for reducing the risk of injury from overworked muscles and improving flexibility. After a strenuous day on the trail, stretching can help muscle cells repair themselves.

How to Stretch

Pick a spot of level ground, free of stones and sticks. Your sleeping bag or pad makes a handy exercise mat. Each of the stretches described in this book should be held for at least 30 seconds at the point of tension, during which time you should feel the tension begin to decrease. Exhale as you lean into the stretch.

Relax and breathe steadily during the stretch. Do not bounce. Bouncing can tear at the muscles and tendons, creating damage that won't be able to heal as you hike. Also, do not overstretch. A small burning feeling is all right, pain is not.

The order of a stretching routine is important. You should always:

Stretch the upper and lower back before stretching your sides.

Stretch your buttocks before stretching your groin.

Stretch your buttocks and calf before stretching your hamstrings.

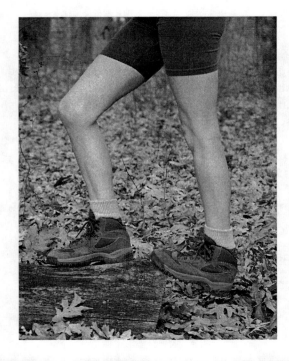

Calf Stretch

Find a rock or stump with a flat top several inches off the ground.

Stand on the rock or stump with your heels hanging off the edge.

Lower both heels until you feel a stretch in your calves.

Raise both heels, then alternately lower your right and then your left heel, stretching each calf for 30 seconds.

Your hiking partner, if you have one, can help you balance.

Please note that while this stretch is helpful, you should use it carefully. It is possible to overstretch the calf and Achilles while doing the calf stretch. In particular, avoid stretching the muscles past the point of natural movement.

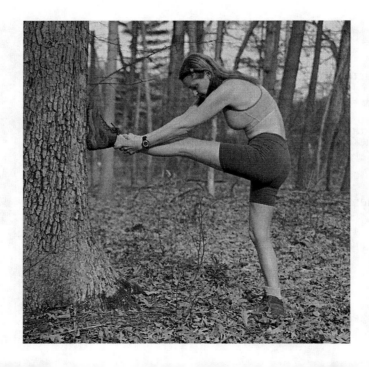

Standing Leg Stretch

Find a tree or big rock. If you use a boulder, its top needs to be at groin height.

Facing the tree or boulder, lift your right leg and place the bottom of your foot against the tree, or rest your heel on the top of the boulder.

Bend forward slowly from the waist and hold the stretch for about 30 seconds.

Repeat the stretch with your left leg.

With your foot in place, turn your body parallel to the tree or boulder.

Bend sideways at the waist, leaning over the outstretched leg.

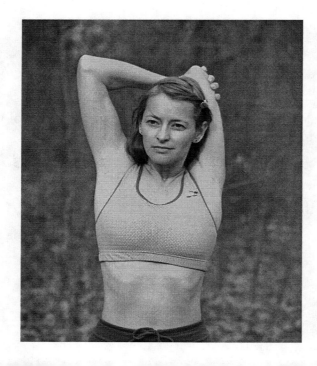

Shoulder Stretch

In a standing position, extend your arms over your head.

Grasp the elbow of your right arm with your left hand. Your right hand is dangling behind your back.

Pull your elbow slowly behind your head, without forcing it.

Repeat the exercise with your left arm.

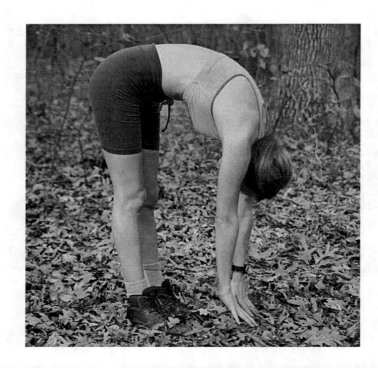

Back Stretch

Stand with your feet about shoulder-width apart.

Slowly bend forward from the waist.

Relax your arms, shoulders, and neck.

Bend until you feel a slight stretch in the backs of your legs. Your back should be rounded.

Once you feel the stretch, hold your position. Do not push yourself to reach the ground.

Bend your knees slightly to relieve pressure on your lower back and return to a standing position.

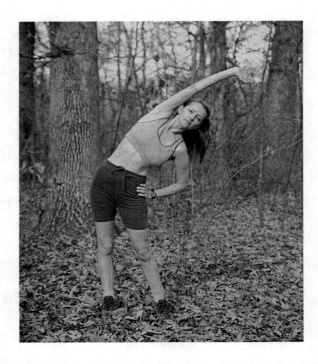

Side Stretch

Stand with your feet about shoulder-width apart.

Keeping your legs straight, place your right hand on your hip and extend your left arm over your head.

Bend toward the right, slowly, until you feel a stretch in your side. Hold.

Repeat the exercise with your left hand on your hip, right arm extended.

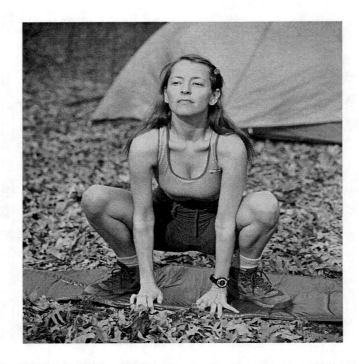

The Squat

Stand with your feet about shoulder-width apart and your toes pointed outward at about 15-degrees.

Lower to a squatting position and place your palms on the ground for balance.

Return to standing, but do not lock your knees, to avoid putting pressure on your lower back.

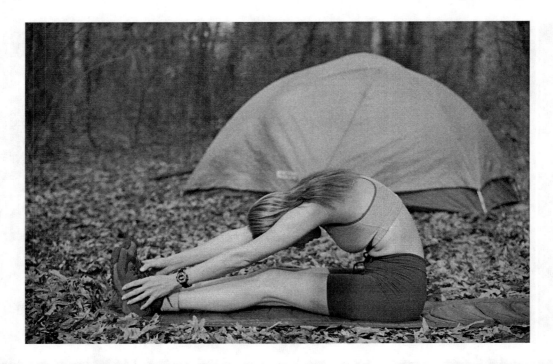

Lower Back Stretch

Sit on the ground (or your sleeping bag or pad) with your legs extended in front of you, flat on the ground, and your feet together.

Flex your toes.

Lean forward, arms extended, reaching for your toes.

Bring your forehead as close to your knees as possible, until you feel a stretch.

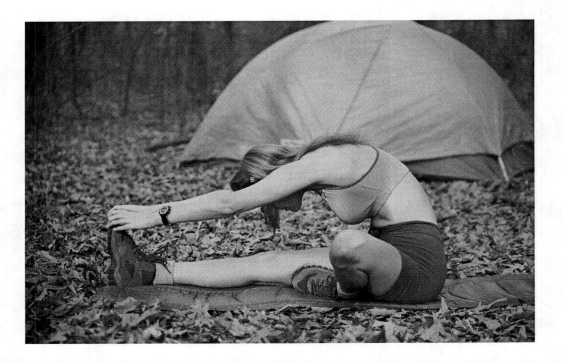

Hamstring Stretch

Sit on the ground (or your sleeping bag or pad) with your legs extended in front of you, flat on the ground.

Pull your right leg toward your body, as you would to sit cross-legged. Place your foot flat against the inside of your left leg.

Lean forward, arms extended. Reach for your toes until you feel a stretch in your left hamstring.

Repeat with your right leg extended and your left leg bent.

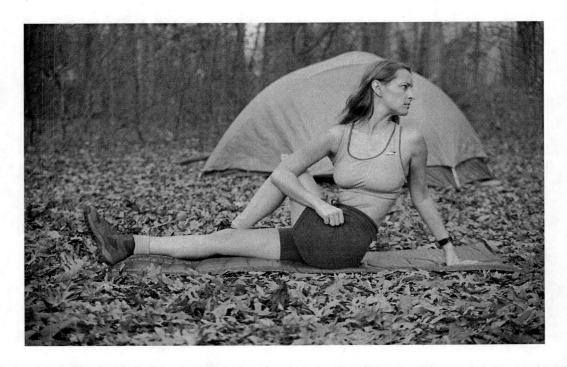

Spinal Stretch

Sit on the ground with your legs extended in front of you.

Bend your left leg and cross it over your right leg; place your left foot on the ground next to your right knee.

Reach your right arm across your left leg and place your right elbow on the outside of your left knee. Your left arm is behind you, keeping your torso erect.

Twist your upper body to the left until you feel a stretch.

Repeat with your left leg outstretched and right leg bent; cross your left arm over your right leg.

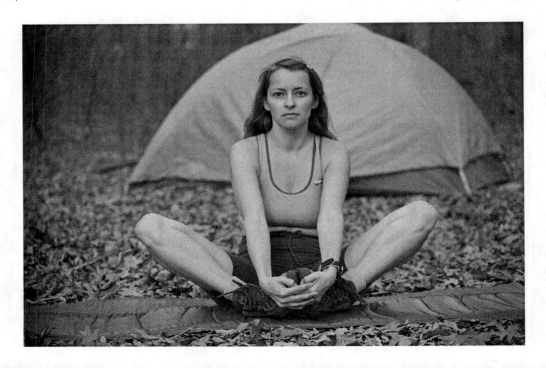

Groin Stretch

Sit on the ground with your legs extended in front of you.

Pull both feet toward you until the soles of your feet are touching.

Gently press your knees toward the ground using your forearms until you feel a stretch in your groin.

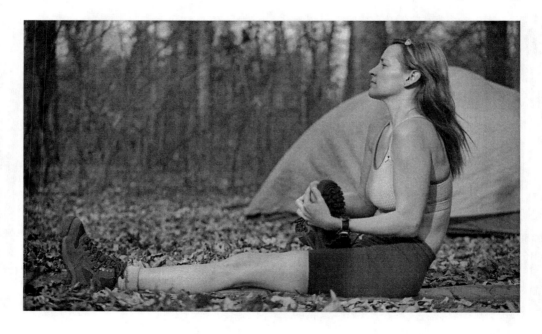

Butt Stretch

Sit on the ground with your legs extended in front of you or lie down on your back.

Grasp your right ankle with both hands, bend your knee, and draw your leg towards your body.

Pull your foot towards your chest until you feel a stretch in your butt.

Repeat with your left leg.

The key to pain relief is a good massage after hiking

Massage

"At the end of the day, when the tent is pitched, is the perfect time for a rejuvenating massage," says Robert Edwards, American Massage Therapy Association spokesperson and co-director of the Somerset School of Massage Therapy in Somerset, New Jersey. Stretching before you exercise can ease the strain on your muscles during the day, and a stretching session after exercise increases flexibility and helps your muscles relax. But the key to pain relief is a good massage after hiking. "After exercise, massage quickens the recovery during a cooldown period," Edwards asserts. "I consider hikers to be athletes, and like all athletes, hikers need to increase circulation and prevent lactic acid from building up in muscles."

Lactic acid and other waste products pool in the blood in your muscles after exercise, and contribute to the sore and jittery feeling in your muscles after a tough day on the trail. "Lactic acid slows down the recovery period after an activity," Edwards says, "but a good massage moves intercellular fluids through the body and allows the spaces created to be filled with oxygen-rich blood and nutrients."

Edwards points out that the benefits of massage—increasing your oxygen supply and purging the body of toxins—can help before you hike as well. "Along with stretching, pre-exercise massage can help prepare the body for activity," he says.

When Not to Massage

There are some times when you should not massage. Avoid massaging directly on a sprained or bruised area; an otherwise helpful massage will only worsen the injury. Treat a sprain or a bruise with RICE—Rest, Ice, Compression, and Elevation. Do not massage hikers who have high blood pressure, a fever, or have been injured during the day. You should also avoid massage with persons who have varicose veins, tumors, rheumatoid arthritis, skin cancer, or an infectious disease, as massage can aggravate these conditions.

Preparing for Massage

You should prepare for massage to make it most effective. Wear loose clothing if you wear clothing at all. The area being massaged should be warm (or your muscles won't relax). It may seem picturesque to have a massage by the side of a mountain pond, but the privacy of your tent makes for a much better atmosphere. A sleeping pad and sleeping bag on the floor of the tent make an ideal massage site—a compromise between a soft and firm surface.

Oil is not essential to massage; however, it can help with certain strokes. Oiled skin eases movement of the hands and helps them slide over body hair. It facilitates the gliding motion of the circulation-enhancing effleurage technique. Effleurage uses long, smooth strokes to push blood toward the heart and increase circulation.

Oil is not essential to massage; however, it can help with certain strokes

Vegetable oils, baby oils, and commercially prepared massage oils all work well. Carry an adequate supply in a plastic 35mm film holder or some other suitable container. Keep a spare towel handy when using oil, in case of spills. The massager should first pour the oil over their hands to warm it, before rubbing it into the skin.

Massage Tips

Be aware that the body's fleshier areas, such as the thighs, can withstand more pressure than places where the bones are closer to the surface, such as the spine. When massaging the back, for example, you should concentrate your efforts on the muscular areas that parallel the spine instead of on the backbone itself.

> *All massage strokes should move from the extremities toward the heart*

All massage strokes should be done working from the extremities toward the heart. Firm massage strokes open up the capillaries and push blood through the veins; you want to work with the natural flow of blood instead of against it.

If you are giving a whole-body massage, using all the techniques in this book in a single session (if time and energy permit), do the back and shoulder strokes in the order shown, then move to the legs and feet. First massage the backs of the legs, then the feet, and last, the fronts of the legs.

Relaxing the muscles is the goal. Work with your partner to learn what feels best. People have different preferences for pressure intensity and some people are more sensitive to certain strokes than others. Encourage your partner to let you know if a stroke is uncomfortable or painful. Listen to your partner's body. Some people need more work in a particular area than these instructions suggest. Allow enough time for a relaxing massage and the results will be more dramatic.

The instructions that follow assume a right-handed person is performing the massage, so if you are left-handed, use the opposite hand than that specified.

What Next?

The massages in this book are a good starting place, but they are only a few of the techniques available. Among the many books on massage, two good sources for further information are *The New Sensual Massage* by Gordon Inkeles and *Massage for Common Ailments* by Sara Thomas. You may also want to try a professional massage before or after your backpacking trip. To find a massage therapist in your area, look in the yellow pages, or contact the American Massage Therapy Association (AMTA) at (847) 864-0123 or www.amtamassage.org.

The back is an easy place to begin massage, because it is very forgiving

Back and Shoulder Massage

The back and shoulders collect stress and tension as you hike. Without massage, they will stay tense for hours or days. The back is an easy place to begin massage, because it is very forgiving. Remember to take it easy on the spinal cord and work on the fleshier portions of the back.

The shoulders move in more complex ways than any other joint, and consequently are more easily stressed than other joints. Take your time when massaging them—loose shoulders will help the whole body relax.

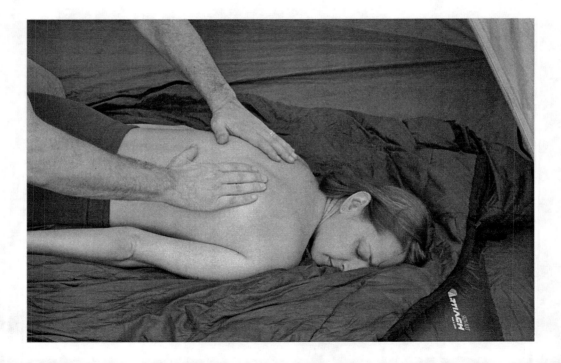

Back and Shoulder Massage
Circulation for the Back

This massage uses long, rhythmic effleurage strokes to get blood flowing and help your partner relax. Keep in contact with your partner's back and shoulders at all times, circling your hands down the sides to begin again.

Have your partner lie face down, then straddle your partner's legs and place your hands on the lower back (where it joins the buttocks).

If you are using oil, pour a little of it in one hand and rub your hands together. Then apply the oil to the back and shoulders in light, even strokes. (The following strokes assume the back and shoulders are oiled.)

Using your fingers and the palm of your hand, push down firmly and slide your hands up your partner's back with the delicate spine between your thumbs.

Continued on page 39

Keep in contact with your partner's back and shoulders at all times

Circulation for the Back continued

Lean into the stroke as you push, conforming your fingers to the shape of the back (shoulders and sides too).

When you have reached the top of the back (or as far as you can reach), glide your hands out and pull back along the sides, continuing to massage as you work back to the top of the buttocks.

As you reach the side of the buttocks, bring your hands together and continue stroking in one smooth motion.

Keep a smooth, even rhythm as you circle the back a half dozen times, pressing deep into the meaty flesh parallel to the spine.

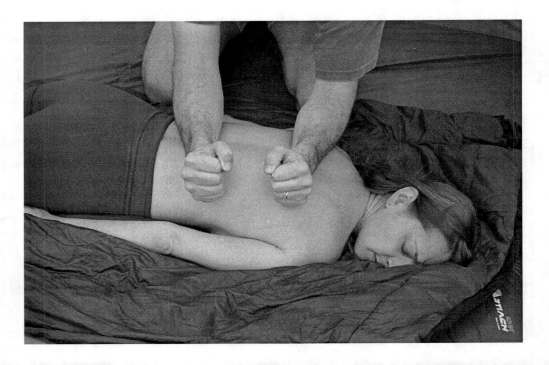

Back and Shoulder Massage
Forearm Stroke

This stroke uses your entire forearm to massage a broad area of your partner's back with a single stroke. The forearm stroke works best with oil.

Kneel beside your partner.

Place your forearms together and lean over until they make contact with the middle of your partner's back.

Press down on the back as you spread your forearms in opposite directions, to the top of the buttocks and to the shoulders.

Pull your forearms together in a smooth motion.

Complete this in/out movement several times.

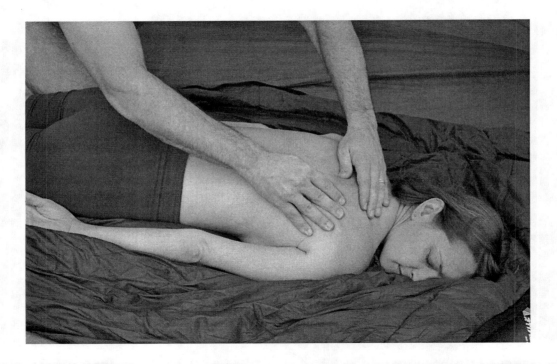

Back and Shoulder Massage
Kneading the Shoulders

To relieve tension in stiff and achy shoulders, try this kneading technique. Spend as much time as necessary in order to loosen tight muscles.

Lay both hands on one of your partner's shoulders.

Use your left hand to push flesh into your right hand.

Pinch the flesh between the thumb and forefinger of your right hand.

Work your way around the shoulder, circling from the base of the shoulder blade up over the top and back around.

Massage one shoulder until the muscles begin to relax and then move to the other.

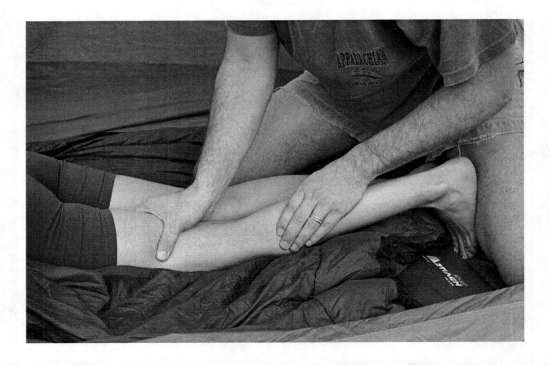

Leg Circulation

Long, steady effleurage strokes on the legs get the blood flowing. Like all effleurage strokes, this leg circulation stroke should be done toward the heart, not toward your feet. If you have limited time for massage, this is the one stroke to use on the legs. This stroke kick-starts the natural self-healing process; it will prepare your partner's legs for other leg massages by getting the blood flowing.

With your partner lying facedown, kneel beside the legs.

If you are using oil, pour a little in one hand and rub your hands together. Then apply the oil to the legs in light even strokes. (The following strokes assume the legs are oiled.)

Cup your hands around one ankle as shown in the photo.

Continued on page 47

Like all effleurage strokes, this leg circulation stroke should be done toward the heart, not toward your feet

Leg Circulation continued

Push your hands up the leg toward the upper thigh with slow, firm strokes.

Alternate hands for each complete full-leg stroke.

Do a dozen full strokes on the back of each leg.

If you are doing a whole body massage, work on the feet next. Then do a dozen full strokes on the front of each leg.

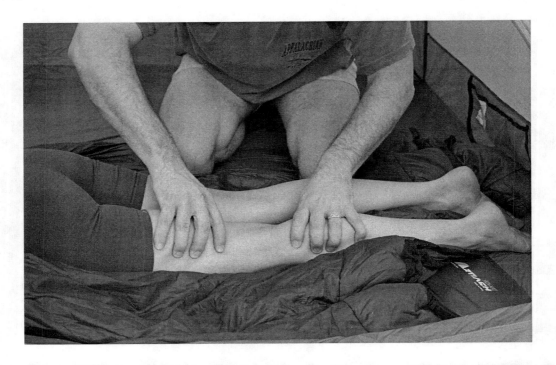

Leg Kneading

A kneading stroke allows you to massage the leg muscles more deeply than the effleurage stroke. Pinching the flesh between your fingers and thumbs continues to push toxins out of the leg muscles and replace them with oxygen-rich blood. As with other strokes, a slow steady pace is most relaxing to your partner.

With your partner lying facedown, grasp the back of the legs with both hands.

Work your way up the legs, from the ankle to the buttocks; squeeze the flesh between your thumb and forefinger, pinching it gently.

As you work your way up the back of the leg, be sure to knead the sides of the leg as well as the top.

Knead the back of each leg several times before moving on to another stroke.

Continued on page 51

A slow steady pace is most relaxing to your partner

Leg Kneading continued

If you are doing a whole body massage, work on the feet next and then the front of the legs.

If you're only massaging the legs, have your partner roll over, then bend one leg at the knee to massage the calf from the front.

Work your way up to the top of the thighs, gently kneading as you go.

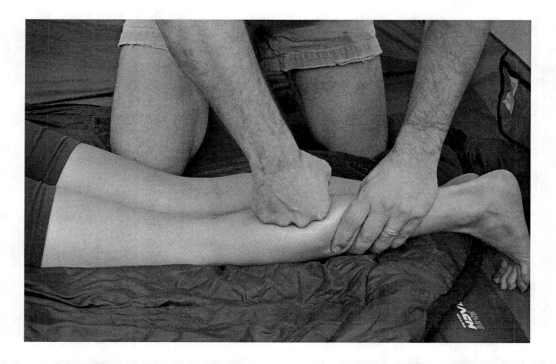

Leg Friction

Friction strokes massage the muscles deeply. This technique works equally well with or without oil. With all friction strokes you should be concerned not with the skin but with the muscles beneath. You'll be able to feel the muscle fibers separate as you press into your partner's legs.

Have your partner lie facedown.

Make a fist with your right hand.

Press firmly into your partner's leg with the front of your fist (as shown); keep your balance with your left hand on the ground or on your partner's leg.

Rotate your fist and feel the muscles moving against the bones. Complete three turns on each spot.

Continued on page 55

*Friction strokes massage
the muscles deeply*

Leg Friction continued

Move your fist up the leg (avoiding the fragile back of the knee), pressing
in at each hand-length along the way to separate the muscle fibers.

*A variation on this stroke is to open your hand and use your fingertips instead
of your fist to press into the muscles.*

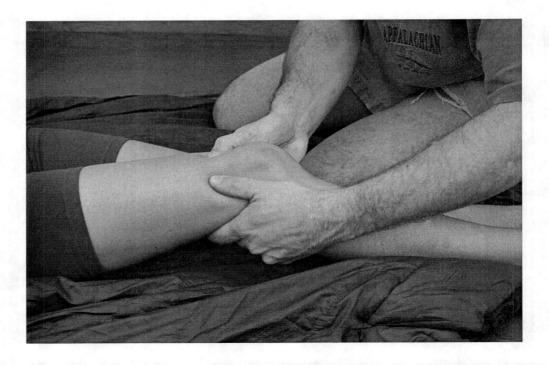

Kneading the Knees

Downhill stretches of trail give your knees a real workout. The complex knee joint is at the center of powerful leg muscles, but requires more delicate treatment than the fleshier thighs. Use your fingertips to knead this important area.

With your partner lying face-up, gently grasp the left knee with both hands.

With small movements, rotate your fingertips and thumbs around the fleshy areas between the bones.

Move your fingers down the both sides of the knee until they meet under the joint; your thumbs stay on top of the leg (as shown). Knead the area just above the knee.

A foot massage relieves stress and helps you relax and get ready for a good night's sleep

Foot Massage

Your feet bear the strain of hiking and backpacking more intensely than any other part of your body. The foot has hundreds of nerve endings packed into a small space. At the end of the day, a foot massage relieves stress and helps you relax and get ready for a good night's sleep.

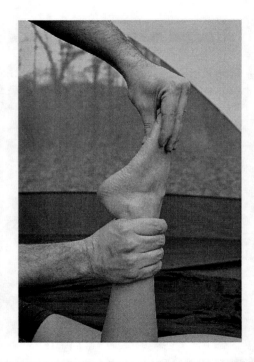

Foot Massage
Rotating the Top of the Foot

The joint in the middle of the foot will not rotate in a complete circle. Work within the natural limitations of the foot without forcing it.

With your partner lying face down, bend one leg at the knee and grasp the ankle firmly in your left hand.

With your right hand, firmly grasp the top of the foot, clamping your hand over the toes.

Pull up to the point of tension.

Rotate the top of the foot in an uneven circle, continuing to pull gently.

Do three full rotations in each direction, pulling outward to create tension as you rotate.

Repeat on the other foot.

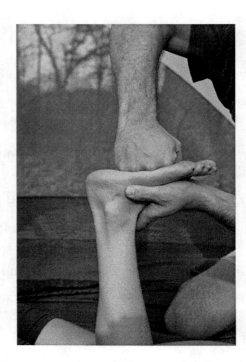

Foot Massage
Knuckle Pressing the Arch

The foot is built to withstand a lot of pressure. You will have to be firm with this maneuver to get the desired effect.

Continue kneeling alongside your partner after rotating the top of the foot and cup your left hand under one foot.

Make your right hand into a fist and push it into the sole of the foot, pushing back on the top of the foot with your other hand.

Rotate the front of your fist back and forth as you continue to press it into the arch.

Repeat on the opposite foot.

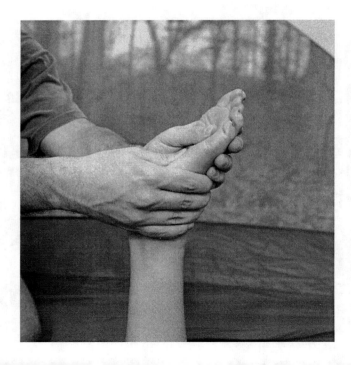

Foot Massage
Thumbing the Foot

Use heavy pressure with your thumbs to stimulate the soles of your partner's feet and ease muscle tension.

With your partner still lying face down, bend one leg at the knee.

Grasp one foot firmly in both hands so that your fingers fit around the top of the foot and your thumbs fall together in the arch.

Push firmly into the sole of your partner's foot.

Walk your thumbs all over the arch, keeping them close together and applying heavy pressure.

Knead the arch from the heels to the toes and back again.

Repeat on the other foot.

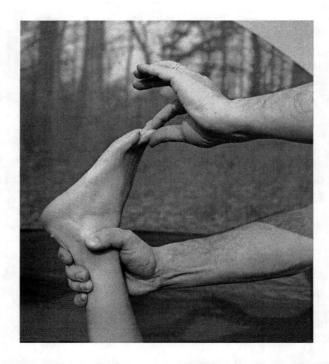

Foot Massage
Massaging the Toes

Toe massage is detail work and you should use gentle pressure with your fingertips on these delicate extremities. Before massaging each toe individually, gently pull it apart from its nearest neighbors until the web of skin between them reaches the point of tension.

Cup the top of your partner's foot in your left hand and take the big toe in your right hand.

Pull the toe out to the point of tension and rotate it three times in each direction.

Repeat this process, massaging each of the nine remaining toes individually. Release your hold on the top of the foot and use your other hand to pull the toes away on either side.

Self-Massage

*E*ven if you don't have a hiking partner (or don't have one you want to massage you), your aching muscles don't have to fend for themselves after a day of hiking or backpacking. Here are a few techniques that you can use on yourself to relieve the physical stress of a day on the trail.

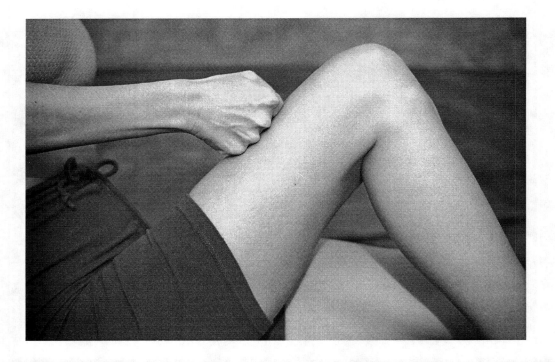

Compression

This technique spreads out your muscle fibers and gets your blood flowing. Use your fingers to compress the middle of your muscle against the underlying bone. Press firmly and rotate the muscles several times in each direction. This technique works well for self-massage on your calves and thighs. For the tops of your thighs, which have a thicker layer of flesh, you may want to use your elbow to compress the muscle, instead of your hands.

Compression is a good technique for a pre-exercise warm-up. Use it before stretching and hiking to get your blood flowing.

This technique works well for self-massage on your calves and thighs

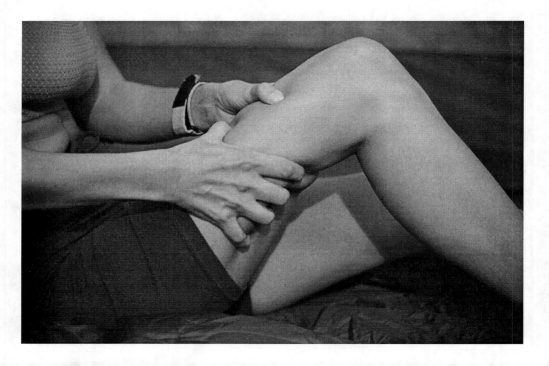

Wringing

This technique works well on the fleshy area just above your knee as well as on your upper thighs.

Grip one thigh firmly in both hands.

Work your hands back and forth from one side of your leg to the other.

Move your hands with the skin, massaging against the grain of the muscle (the muscles run lengthwise—you are rubbing side-to-side) to create a warm feeling deep under the skin.

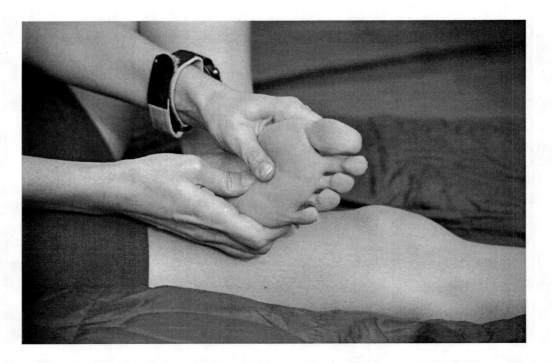

Thumbing Your Feet

In a sitting position, cross one leg over the other just above the knee so that your ankle is resting on your thigh.

Grasp one foot firmly in both hands so that your fingers fit around the top of your foot and your thumbs fall together in the arch.

Push firmly with your thumbs into the sole of the foot.

Walk your thumbs all over your arch, keeping them close together and applying heavy pressure.

Knead the arch from the heels to the toes and back again.

Repeat on your other foot.

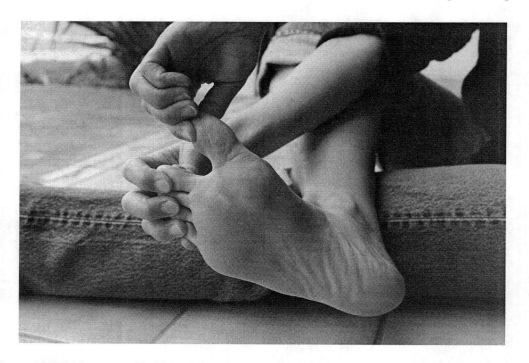

Massaging Your Toes

Gently pull each toe apart from its nearest neighbors until the web of skin between them reaches the point of tension.

Cup the top of the foot in one hand and take the big toe in the other.

Pull the toe out to the point of tension and rotate it three times in each direction.

Repeat this process, massaging each of the nine remaining toes individually.

Over 30 Years of Outdoor Expertise from Wilderness Press!

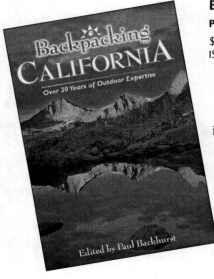

Backpacking California
PAUL BACKHURST, ED.

$21.95, 1st edition, 520 pages, 6 x 9, softbound
ISBN 0-89997-286-1   UPC 7-19609-97286-0

A compendium of the best California backpacks.

Here are 62 trips by 17 Wilderness Press authors, each in a unique and personal style. Trips range from overnights to two-week treks in the Coast Ranges from Mexico to Oregon, the Sierra Nevada, the Cascades, and the Warner Mountains.

Routes include portions of the Pacific Crest Trail, the High Sierra Trail, and the John Muir Trail. Each trip includes a complete description; a trail map showing the trailhead, route, and terminus; campsites; mileage; and an at-a-glance hiking difficulty chart.

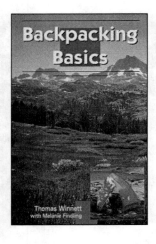

Backpacking Basics

WINNETT & FINDLING

$9.95, 4th edition
134 pages, 5 x 7½,
softbound
ISBN 0-89997-172-5
UPC 7-19609-97172-6

Take the mystery out of your first backpacking trip. Learn all you need to know for a comfortable, safe, and enjoyable adventure: when and where to go, what to take, how much you can comfortably carry, and how to pack.

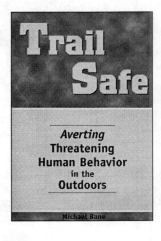

Trail Safe

Averting Threatening Human Behavior in the Outdoors

MICHAEL BANE

$14.95, 1st edition
176 pages, 5½ x 8½,
softbound
ISBN 0-89997-264-0
UPC 7-19609-97264-8

Strengthen your confidence in the backcountry. Here is practical advice that helps you use your awareness, intuition, and fear to protect yourself on our outdoor adventures. Author Michael Bane provides essential tips on how to stay safe.

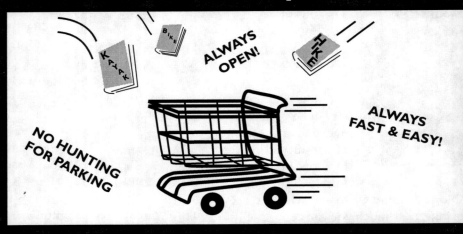